From Diagnosis to Recovery

A Parent's Survival Guide to Support Guillain-Barré Syndrome in Children

Dr. Travis R. Hill

Table of Content

INTRODUCTION

Guillain-Barré Syndrome (GBS) has an intriguing history that dates back to the 19th century. French physician Jean Baptiste Octave Landry first wrote about it in 1859.

He identified it as a form of ascending paralysis, characterized by symptoms that begin in the legs and move upward through the body. Due to Landry's initial reports, the condition was initially known as Landry's paralysis.

In 1916, French neurologists Georges Guillain, Jean-Alexandre Barre, and Andre Strohl conducted additional studies, which significantly advanced our understanding of the syndrome.

They discovered that patients exhibiting symptoms similar to Landry's paralysis had elevated protein levels in their cerebrospinal fluid, a key diagnostic marker that distinguished it from other neurological disorders. This discovery marked a significant advancement in diagnosing as well as comprehending the syndrome.

Landry's earlier study was acknowledged when Guillain and Barré published a report in 1919 detailing a case of deadly illness. Despite André Strohl's contributions to the research, his name was not included in the commonly used term for the condition, which became widely known as Guillain-Barré Syndrome. In some instances, it is also referred to as Guillain-Barré-Strohl Syndrome, reflecting Strohl's involvement.

Since these early discoveries, the understanding and treatment of Guillain-Barré Syndrome have evolved considerably. Medical technology and research advances have improved diagnostic techniques, leading to more accurate and timely identification of the condition.

Today, GBS is recognized as an autoimmune disorder, with treatment strategies focused on managing symptoms and supporting recovery through therapies such as plasmapheresis and intravenous immunoglobulin (IVIG).

Ongoing research continues to explore the underlying mechanisms of GBS and its potential links to infections and other triggers, enhancing our understanding of this complex syndrome. By studying its history and developments, we gain valuable insights into the progress made in treating and managing Guillain-Barré Syndrome, providing hope for those affected by this condition.

The peripheral nerve system is impacted by the uncommon autoimmune disease known as Guillain-Barré syndrome. Its severity can vary from mild to extreme, with the most serious cases leading to muscle paralysis and potentially life-threatening complications with breathing and swallowing.

While this condition can impact individuals of any age, it is slightly more prevalent in adults and tends to occur more often in males. This autoimmune condition arises when the body's immune system mistakenly attacks healthy nerves, leading to a range of symptoms that can vary significantly from one person to another.

Understanding the basics of GBS is the first step in supporting your child through this challenging experience. Guillain-Barré Syndrome is characterized by the rapid onset of muscle weakness and, in some cases, paralysis.

This weakness typically begins in the legs and spreads to the upper body, but it can affect different areas in different individuals. GBS can progress quickly, with symptoms worsening for days to weeks. While the exact cause of GBS remains unknown, it often follows an infection, such as a respiratory or gastrointestinal illness. In rare cases, GBS can be triggered by surgery or vaccinations.

The syndrome is considered a medical emergency because of the potential for rapid progression and the risk of severe complications. Early recognition and treatment are crucial to improve outcomes and reduce the likelihood of long-term effects.

As a parent facing a diagnosis of Guillain-Barré syndrome in your child, it can be an overwhelming and frightening experience. This guide aims to provide you with the information, support, and resources needed to navigate this challenging journey.

From understanding the initial symptoms and navigating the healthcare system to supporting your child through treatment and recovery, this book provides you with the knowledge and self-assurance needed to stand up for your child's health and welfare.

In the following pages, we will explore the various aspects of Guillain-Barré syndrome, from diagnosis to recovery, offering practical advice and personal stories from other parents who have faced similar challenges. Our goal is to provide a comprehensive resource that not only explains the medical aspects of the condition but also addresses the emotional and psychological impact on both your child and your family.

By learning more about Guillain-Barré syndrome and connecting with others who have experienced it, you can find hope and strength in the shared journey toward recovery. This book is here to guide you every step of the way, offering support and encouragement as you navigate the journey ahead.

CHAPTER 1

Getting the Diagnosis

Parents can feel overwhelmed when their child is diagnosed with Guillain-Barré Syndrome (GBS). Understanding the diagnostic process can allow you to navigate the healthcare system better and advocate for the needs of your child.

This chapter will walk you through the process of diagnosing GBS, from identifying early symptoms to the tests and procedures utilized by healthcare experts.

Identifying Early Symptoms

The first step in diagnosing GBS is to identify the early symptoms, which usually appear unexpectedly and progress quickly. Early warning indications include:

- **Muscle weakness:** This typically starts in the legs and might extend to the arms and the upper body.

- **Tingling or Numbness:** A feeling of pins and needles in the hands and feet.

- **Difficulty Walking:** Leg weakness can result in uneven walking or the inability to walk.

- **Reflex loss:** Decreased reflexes in the knees and ankles.

- **Pain:** Aching or cramping, usually in the back or limbs.

In severe cases, symptoms may worsen to include breathing problems, swallowing, and speaking. If your child shows any of these symptoms, get medical assistance immediately.

Medical Tests and Procedures

Once GBS is suspected, several tests and assessments are performed to confirm the diagnosis. The most popular diagnostic tools are:

- **Neurological Examination:** A neurologist will thoroughly examine your child's reflexes, muscle strength, and coordination to look for symptoms of nerve damage.

- **Lumbar Puncture (Spinal Tap):** This procedure includes taking a sample of cerebrospinal fluid (CSF) from the lower back to detect increased protein levels, which are common in GBS.

- **Electromyography (EMG) and Nerve Conduction Studies (NCS):** These tests detect muscle electrical activity and nerve signal transmission speed, which aids in identifying nerve damage and distinguishing between demyelinating and axonal forms of GBS.

- **Blood Tests:** While no particular blood test can identify GBS, tests can be used to rule out other illnesses and look for infections that could cause the syndrome.

Communicate with Healthcare Providers

Solid interaction with your child's healthcare team is critical for a prompt and correct diagnosis. Here are some suggestions for working with medical professionals:

- **Prepare for Appointments**: Document any symptoms your kid has had, including when they started and progression. Note any recent illnesses or infections, as well as any relevant family history.

- **Ask questions:** Feel free to seek clarification on the diagnosis, tests, or treatment alternatives. Understanding the facts allows you to make informed decisions about your child's care.

- **Seek a Second Opinion:** See another doctor for a second opinion if you are worried about the diagnosis or treatment plan.

- **Stay Informed:** Learn about GBS from credible sources to better understand the illness and the reasoning behind medical decisions.

Early detection and intervention are crucial for controlling Guillain-Barré Syndrome. Prompt medical care can help lessen the intensity of symptoms, prevent complications, and increase the likelihood of complete recovery. Once a diagnosis has been confirmed, your child's healthcare team will collaborate with you to create a customized treatment plan.

CHAPTER 2

Pathophysiology of Guillain-Barré Syndrome

The pathophysiological processes that lead to Guillain-Barré Syndrome (GBS) are intricate and involve an autoimmune response. It is believed that the immune system mistakenly targets the peripheral nerves due to the presence of infectious agents such as bacteria or viruses that share structural similarities with components of the peripheral nerve cells.

This molecular mimicry causes the immune system to attack both the infectious agents and the body's nerve cells. This misguided immune response results in inflammation and the destruction of the myelin sheath, the fatty layer that insulates nerve fibers and facilitates the transmission of electrical signals.

Myelin loss causes paralysis, numbness, and even muscle weakness. In severe cases, the axons, which are the core components of nerves responsible for conducting impulses, may also be damaged.

Guillain-Barré Syndrome can be categorized into various subtypes based on pathophysiological and clinical characteristics. It is often classified into demyelinating and axonal types.

The most prevalent type is Acute Inflammatory Demyelinating Polyneuropathy (AIDP), which destroys the myelin sheath. Axonal variants include Acute Motor Axonal Neuropathy (AMAN) and Acute Motor and Sensory Axonal Neuropathy (AMSAN), which primarily affect the axons themselves.

Miller Fisher Syndrome, a rare form of GBS that develops quickly, is distinguished by three primary symptoms: areflexia (absence of reflexes), ataxia (loss of coordination), and ophthalmoplegia (weakness in the eye muscles resulting in double vision).

Understanding these pathophysiological mechanisms is crucial for diagnosing and treating Guillain-Barré Syndrome effectively, allowing for more targeted therapeutic approaches and improved outcomes for those affected by this condition.

CHAPTER 3

Treatment and Recovery

Guillain-Barré Syndrome (GBS) treatment consists of both immediate and long-term recovery. Understanding the variety of options for treatment and stages of recovery will help you support your child effectively during this difficult time.

Treatment Options

After a GBS diagnosis is confirmed, the focus shifts towards symptom management and complication prevention. Treatment is often administered in a hospital setting, where your kid can receive the appropriate care and monitoring. Here are the primary treatment approaches:

1. **Hospitalization and Acute Care**

   - Monitoring and Support: Your child will most likely be admitted to a hospital and constantly watched for any changes in symptoms. This includes regular monitoring of respiration, heart rate, and blood pressure.

   - Respiratory Support: In severe instances where muscle weakness makes breathing difficult, mechanical ventilation may be required.

2. **Medications and therapies**

   - Plasmapheresis (Plasma Exchange): This is a treatment in which the plasma portion of the blood is removed and replaced to minimize antibodies that assault peripheral nerves.

   - Intravenous Immunoglobulin (IVIG): High doses of immunoglobulin are supplied intravenously to help block the dangerous antibodies that cause nerve injury.

- Pain management: Pain relievers and anti-inflammatory medications can help manage the discomfort and pain caused by GBS.

3. Managing pain and discomfort

- Physical Therapy: Gentle exercises and physiotherapy can help keep muscles strong and flexible, preventing stiffness in the muscles and contractures.

- Occupational Therapy: Occupational Therapists can help people adjust their daily routines to accommodate physical limitations and encourage independence.

The Recovery Process

Recovery from GBS varies greatly from person to person, depending on the severity of the condition and how the individual responds to treatment. Here is a summary of the recovery stages:

1. Understanding Recovery Stages

- The acute phase, in which symptoms worsen, usually lasts a few weeks. This is followed by an indefinite period, during which symptoms stabilize.

- The recovery phase involves progressive improvement in strength and function. Recovery can take weeks or months, and some people need a year or more to fully recover.

2. **Physical and Occupational Therapy**

- Rehabilitation Programs: Personalized rehabilitation programs are critical for restoring strength and mobility. These could include activities that improve balance, coordination, and endurance.

- Assistive Devices: Temporary usage of assistive devices, such as walkers or braces, may be required to support mobility during the rehabilitation process.

3. **Emotional and Psychological Support**

- **Counseling and Support Groups:** Emotional and psychological support can be extremely beneficial in recovery. Counseling and support groups for your child and family members can offer helpful encouragement and coping strategies.

- **Encourage Resilience:** Keeping a positive attitude and having attainable goals might help your child stay motivated during the rehabilitation process.

As a parent, you play an important role in helping your child during treatment and recovery. Many children can recover completely from Guillain-Barré Syndrome with the proper treatment and support.

CHAPTER 4

Causes and Risk Factors of Guillain-Barré Syndrome

GBS, also known as Guillain-Barré Syndrome, is an autoimmune disorder; however, the precise cause of this condition is not completely understood.

Several factors can increase the risk of developing GBS, with recent infections being one of the most significant triggers. Understanding these factors can help identify and manage the condition.

Potential Causes

1. Autoimmune Reaction: GBS occurs when the immune system mistakenly attacks the nerves. This response is thought to happen when certain infections or medical events alter the nerve cells, causing the immune system to perceive them as threats.

In Acute Inflammatory Demyelinating Polyneuropathy (AIDP), the most common type of GBS, the myelin sheath (the protective covering of nerves) is damaged, disrupting the transmission of signals between the brain and muscles. Sometimes, the axon, the core of the nerve, may also be damaged.

2. Infections and Illnesses: Many cases of GBS follow an infection, such as a respiratory or gastrointestinal illness. About two-thirds of individuals with GBS report having experienced diarrhea or respiratory symptoms in the days or weeks preceding the onset of neurological symptoms.

3. Vaccinations and Medical Events: Although rare, some vaccines and medical procedures have been associated with GBS. It's crucial to discuss vaccination history and recent medical events with healthcare providers.

4. Genetic Factors: While GBS is not hereditary, certain genetic factors may increase susceptibility to the syndrome.

Risk Factors

Anyone is vulnerable to contracting GBS; however, certain factors can make the risk higher:

1. Age and Gender: GBS is slightly more common in adults, particularly those over 50, and is more frequently observed in males than females.

2. Infections: Several infectious agents are linked to the development of GBS, including:

- Campylobacter jejuni: A bacteria commonly found in undercooked poultry and considered the most common trigger.

- Viruses: Such as the influenza virus, COVID-19, cytomegalovirus, Epstein-Barr virus, Zika virus, and hepatitis A, B, C, and E.

- Human immunodeficiency virus (HIV) is the virus that causes AIDS.

- Mycoplasma pneumonia.

3. Surgery and Trauma: Some individuals develop GBS following surgical procedures or traumatic events, although the reasons for this are not entirely clear.

4. Illnesses and Medical Conditions:

- Hodgkin's lymphoma has been associated with an increased risk of GBS.

5. Vaccinations: There have been rare instances where certain COVID-19 vaccines (specifically those from Johnson & Johnson and AstraZeneca) have been linked to GBS.

While exposure to these factors can increase the likelihood of developing GBS, it is still unclear why only some people develop the syndrome following such triggers. Understanding these risk factors can help in the early identification and management of GBS, leading to more effective treatment and recovery.

CHAPTER 5

Signs and Symptoms

Recognizing the signs and symptoms of Guillain-Barré Syndrome (GBS) early can be crucial for timely medical intervention. The symptoms typically progress over hours to days, and understanding them can help ensure prompt treatment and support. Here is a comprehensive overview of the common signs and symptoms associated with GBS:

Early Symptoms

1. Muscle Weakness: Often the first noticeable symptom, muscle weakness usually starts in the legs and can progressively spread upwards to the arms and upper body.

2. Tingling Sensations: Affected individuals may experience numbness or tingling in the hands and feet, which can extend to other areas of the body.

3. Difficulty Walking: Weakness in the legs can make walking difficult or impossible, impacting mobility and balance.

4. Pain: Some individuals report nerve pain, which can be severe and is often most intense in the shoulder girdle, back, buttocks, and thighs. This pain may be described as aching or throbbing.

5. Reflex Loss: Diminished or absent reflexes in the arms and legs can be indicative of GBS.

Progressing Symptoms

As GBS progresses, additional symptoms may develop, including:

1. Difficulty Breathing and Swallowing: Severe cases can affect the muscles involved in breathing and swallowing. This may result in difficulties with these functions, which might demand immediate medical attention, including the use of mechanical ventilation.

2. Facial and Cranial Nerve Involvement: Common complaints include:

- Face drooping: This could look like Bell's palsy.

- Diplopia (Double Vision).

- Dysarthria (Difficulty Speaking).

- Dysphagia (Difficulty Swallowing).

- Ophthalmoplegia (Eye Muscle Weakness).

- Pupillary Disturbances.

3. Sensory Changes: Paresthesias, or abnormal sensations such as "pins and needles," often start in the toes and fingertips, progressing upwards but generally not extending beyond the wrists or ankles.

4. Coordination and Mobility Issues: An unsteady gait, difficulty walking upstairs, and problems with coordination may be present.

In some cases, GBS can lead to severe complications, including:

1. Paralysis: Progressive paralysis of the legs, arms, or face can occur, potentially affecting chewing and swallowing. Around 20 to 30 percent of individuals may experience paralysis of chest muscles, which can lead to ventilatory failure and necessitate respiratory support.

2. Autonomic Changes: These changes can include:

- Tachycardia (Rapid Heart Rate).

- Bradycardia (Slow Heart Rate).

- Facial Flushing.

- Paroxysmal Hypertension (Intermittent High Blood Pressure).

- Orthostatic Hypotension (Decrease in Blood Pressure While Standing).

- Anhidrosis and/or Diaphoresis (Reduced or Excessive Sweating).

- Urinary Retention.

3. Respiratory Complaints: Symptoms may include:

- Dyspnea on Exertion: Breathlessness During Activities.

- Shortness of Breath.

- Difficulty Swallowing.

- Slurred Speech.

The typical patient with GBS, particularly Acute Inflammatory Demyelinating Polyneuropathy (AIDP), often presents 2-4 weeks after a relatively mild respiratory or gastrointestinal illness.

Initial complaints include finger dysesthesias and proximal muscle weakness in the lower extremities, which can progress to involve the arms, trunk, cranial nerves, and respiratory muscles.

Understanding these symptoms can help in recognizing the condition early and seeking appropriate medical care.

CHAPTER 6

Living with Guillain-Barré Syndrome and Supporting Your Child

Coping With Guillain-Barré Syndrome

Living with Guillain-Barré Syndrome (GBS) can be difficult for both the kid and their parents. The path taken from diagnosis to recovery entails dealing with medical symptoms, emotional stress, and practical problems. Here's an outline for navigating life with GBS:

1. Understanding the Condition:

- Educate yourself about GBS to better support your child. Knowing about the illness allows you to anticipate needs and make informed decisions about care and treatment.

- Maintain open communication with your child's medical staff. Regular updates and talks about your child's progress, as well as any changes in symptoms, can help you adjust the treatment plan as needed.

2. Managing Symptoms and Treatment:

- Medication and Therapies: Adhere to the prescribed treatment plan, including medications, physical therapy, and additional interventions. Treatment adherence is critical for recovery and symptom management.

- Physical Therapy: Perform physical therapy as advised. It might be critical in helping your child regain strength and mobility. Be patient, and encourage your child to think positively about their growth.

3. Emotional Support:

- Reassurance: Offer emotional support and comfort to your child. Dealing with GBS can be terrifying, so provide comfort and understanding.

- Counseling: You might consider obtaining counseling or joining a support group for both your child and yourself. Connecting with others who have faced similar issues can offer emotional support and practical help.

4. Daily Living Adjustments:

- Home Modifications: Adjust your home to meet your child's physical demands. This could include adding grab bars, ramps, or other accessible measures.

- Assistive Devices: Wheelchairs, walkers, and other mobility aids can help your kid navigate daily activities.

5. Monitor and follow-up:

- Schedule and attend monthly follow-up appointments to assess your child's health and progress. Keeping up with medical appointments helps to ensure that any concerns are handled as soon as possible.

- Emergency Plan: Prepare for future emergencies by developing an action plan. Learn the warning signals of serious complications and how to respond if your child's condition worsens.

Supporting your child's GBS journey requires both practical and emotional care. Here are some ideas to ensure your child gets the help they need:

1. Emotional Encouragement:

- Positive Reinforcement: Recognize little triumphs and progress, no matter how minor they appear. Positive reinforcement increases confidence and motivation.

- Open Dialogue: Encourage your youngster to communicate their emotions and worries. Listen actively and reassure them that you are there to help.

2. Practical Assistance:

- Provide daily care, including personal care, mobility, and domestic tasks as needed. Make sure that your child is comfortable and supported in their everyday routines.

- Educational Support: If your child attends school, engage with teachers and staff about their condition. Collaborate to develop a suitable plan for their education and accommodations.

3. Involving the Family:

- Family Roles: Involve family members in caring. Sharing chores can help reduce stress and ensure that your child receives complete care.

- Family Activities: Plan family activities that are both entertaining and appropriate for your child's condition. Maintaining a feeling of normalcy helps boost your child's mood and make them feel involved.

4. Caregivers' Self-Care:

- Stress Management: Caregivers often face high demands. Take time for self-care and seek help when necessary. Your well-being is critical to providing excellent care for your children.

- Seek support: Don't be afraid to ask for support from friends, family, or professionals. Other people's help can make a big difference in dealing with the problems of caregiving.

By addressing both the practical and emotional aspects of living with Guillain-Barré Syndrome, you can help your child recover and improve their overall well-being.

CHAPTER 7

Long-Term Outlook and Management

The long-term prognosis for children with Guillain-Barré Syndrome (GBS) is generally good, with many achieving a complete recovery. However, the healing process might vary greatly depending on the severity of the illness and the individual's response to treatment.

Understanding the likely course of the ailment and the management options involved is critical for both caregivers and healthcare professionals. Following the immediate aftermath of GBS, the focus changes to rehabilitation and recovery. Physical therapy is a critical component of this process, helping children restore muscle strength, movement, and coordination.

Customized physical therapy regimens are developed to meet each child's demands while changing as their condition develops.

The recovery process might be gradual, and continued physical therapy may be required for several months or even years, depending on the severity of the initial symptoms and the individual's progression.

Regular follow-up visits with healthcare providers are essential for monitoring the child's progress and addressing any potential issues. These appointments allow for the evaluation of recovery, adjustments to treatment programs, and early intervention if new symptoms or difficulties occur.

Caregivers must keep open communication with the healthcare staff, offering regular updates on the child's status and expressing any concerns or changes in symptoms.

While most children with GBS recover completely, others may endure persistent symptoms such as moderate weakness, sensory abnormalities, or weariness. Long-term management for these children may need more assistance and changes to their daily routines.

Occupational therapy can help children overcome functional limits and improve their quality of life. In some circumstances, children may require continuous care from professionals such as neurologists or rehabilitation therapists to successfully address and manage these persistent problems.

Emotional and psychological support are also important aspects of long-term management. The effects of GBS on a child's physical ability and daily life can be upsetting and emotionally taxing.

Consistent encouragement, reassurance, and opportunity for the youngster to express their emotions are critical. Counsellors, psychologists, and support groups can help you navigate the emotional components of the condition and retain a positive view.

Parents and caregivers should be prepared for relapses and complications, which are uncommon. Being proactive in monitoring the child's status and keeping to follow-up plans ensures that any potential difficulties are handled as soon as possible.

It is also critical to stay current on GBS and its therapy, as advances in treatment and understanding of the syndrome may affect long-term care methods.

In addition to medical and therapeutic care, practical adaptations in daily living may be required. This could include changing the living environment to accommodate any physical restrictions or utilizing assistive equipment to promote mobility and independence.

Collaborating with educational specialists to build a supportive school environment can also be advantageous in terms of meeting the child's educational needs and providing necessary modifications.

Overall, while recovering from Guillain-Barré Syndrome can be a lengthy and difficult process, with the correct support and care, most children are capable of recovering their prior levels of activity and quality of life.

A complete approach that includes medical treatment, physical and emotional support, and practical modifications is essential for getting the best potential results. By keeping involved in the recovery process and maintaining a positive, proactive attitude, families can assist their children in navigating the hurdles of GBS and emerging stronger on the other side.

CHAPTER 8

Freddie Freeman's Experience and Other Survivor

Personal stories from families who have faced Guillain-Barré Syndrome (GBS) offer valuable perspectives and encouragement. One family's experience with their young child, Catherine, highlights the emotional and practical challenges of GBS.

After Catherine was diagnosed post-flu, her parents felt overwhelmed by the rapid progression of her symptoms. Seeking support from other families and joining online communities provided them with crucial advice and hope.

Catherine's recovery involved intensive physical therapy, which was both demanding and rewarding. Her family celebrated each milestone, from regaining basic mobility to walking again. They made home modifications, such as installing grab bars, to support her progress and ensure safety.

Catherine and her family had emotional challenges throughout their journey. Open communication and professional counseling played essential roles in managing stress and maintaining resilience. They learned to navigate the ups and downs of recovery by staying positive and focusing on their child's achievements.

As Catherine's condition improved, her family adapted to their new normal and used their experience to raise awareness about GBS. They participated in fundraising events and shared their story to support others facing similar challenges.

Their journey demonstrates the importance of community support, adaptability, and a positive outlook. It shows that while GBS can be a difficult path, it is also one filled with growth, connection, and hope, offering a beacon of encouragement for others navigating the condition.

Another notable example is that of Freddie Freeman, the renowned baseball player, and his wife Chelsea, who are facing a challenging journey with their 3-year-old son, Maximus. Recently diagnosed with GBS, Maximus's condition has brought significant emotional and practical challenges to the Freeman family.

GBS, a rare and serious neurological disorder, occurs when the immune system mistakenly attacks the nerves, leading to muscle weakness, numbness, and sometimes paralysis. It can be triggered by a viral or bacterial infection, and its progression can be unpredictable.

Maximus was hospitalized for over a week, receiving intensive care and treatment from medical professionals. Throughout this difficult time, Freddie and Chelsea have been by his side, offering unwavering love and support.

The baseball community and fans have rallied around the Freeman family, providing words of encouragement, prayers, and well-wishes. Freddie and Chelsea have expressed profound gratitude for the outpouring of support, which has been a beacon of hope during their challenging journey.

Fortunately, Maximus has recently returned home and continues his recovery process. His parents remain dedicated to ensuring he receives the necessary treatment and therapy to overcome GBS.

Freddie Freeman has been candid about the emotional toll this experience has taken on their family. Despite the challenges, they stay hopeful and committed to supporting Maximus every step of the way.

The Freeman family's tenacity and strength in the face of difficulties inspire many others. Their journey underscores the importance of community support and the power of staying hopeful, as they navigate the challenges of GBS together.

CHAPTER 9

Key Points and Helpful Tips

Understanding Guillain-Barré Syndrome (GBS)

1. Nature of the Condition: Guillain-Barré Syndrome (GBS) is a rare but serious disorder that affects the peripheral nerves. It is typically short-term but can be life-threatening, and it can occur in any child.

2. Potential Causes: The precise cause of GBS is not fully known, but it is believed to be an autoimmune disorder. This suggests that the immune system of the body unintentionally attacks the nerve cells.

GBS may develop following a viral infection, surgery, injury, or, rarely, as a reaction to a vaccine. Most children with GBS experience symptoms a few days to weeks after having diarrhea or a respiratory illness.

3. Symptoms: GBS can cause muscle weakness, pain, and temporary paralysis affecting the face, chest, legs, and swallowing muscles. Symptoms may include reduced sensation or pain in the fingers and toes and weakness in the arms or legs. If the muscles responsible for breathing and swallowing become paralyzed, it can lead to severe complications such as breathing difficulties, choking, and, if untreated, death.

4. Treatment and Recovery: There isn't a specific treatment for GBS at the moment. While it may resolve on its own, the condition can be life-threatening, requiring intensive care in a hospital setting. Most children diagnosed with GBS make a full recovery, often starting within a few days to weeks after treatment begins.

Maximizing Your Child's Healthcare Visits

Take into account the tips that follow to make the best possible use of your child's doctor visits:

1. Prepare for the Visit:

- Clarify Objectives: Understand the aim of the visit and your desired outcomes.

- Prepare Questions: Write down any questions you have about your child's condition, treatment options, and next steps.

2. During the Visit:

- Document Key Information: Note the new diagnosis, any new medications, treatments, or tests recommended, and any instructions provided by the healthcare provider.

- Understand Prescriptions: Ask about the purpose of any new medications or treatments, their expected benefits, and potential side effects.

- Explore Alternatives: Inquire if there are other treatment options available for your child's condition.

3. Understanding Tests and Procedures:

- Ask About Recommendations: Find out why a test or procedure is recommended and what the results could indicate.

- Consider Consequences: Understand what might happen if your child does not follow through with the prescribed medications or tests.

4. Follow-Up Care:

- Track Appointments: Note the date, time, and purpose of any follow-up visits.

- Emergency Contact: Know how to contact your child's healthcare provider after office hours in case of emergencies or urgent questions.

By staying informed and organized, you can actively participate in your child's care and support their journey through Guillain-Barré Syndrome more effectively.

Conclusion

Guillain-Barré Syndrome (GBS) is a rare and complex condition that presents significant challenges for both those affected and their families. Throughout this book, we have explored the intricacies of GBS—from its symptoms and diagnosis to its treatment and long-term management.

We've delved into the personal stories of families who have faced this formidable disorder, including the journey of Freddie Freeman and his son Maximus, whose experience has shed light on the profound emotional and practical challenges of living with GBS.

The path through Guillain-Barré Syndrome is often fraught with uncertainty and difficulty, but it is also marked by hope, resilience, and the power of support.

Early diagnosis and treatment are crucial, and understanding the symptoms and progression of the syndrome can make a significant difference in outcomes.

The stories of those who have navigated this journey emphasize the importance of perseverance, community, and the unwavering support of loved ones.

For families facing a diagnosis of GBS, the road ahead may seem daunting, but it is navigable with the right resources, support, and care. The advancements in medical treatment and the dedicated efforts of healthcare professionals offer hope for recovery and improvement.

The resilience demonstrated by families, coupled with the support from communities and the broader public, provides a beacon of encouragement for those on this challenging path.

As we conclude this book, we hope that the information and personal insights shared will serve as a valuable resource for parents, caregivers, and anyone affected by Guillain-Barré Syndrome.

By fostering a deeper understanding of the condition and highlighting the experiences of those who have walked this path, we aim to offer support and hope to those facing similar struggles. Remember, while the journey with GBS may be challenging, it is also one that can be navigated with courage, community, and an unwavering commitment to recovery.

Appendices

Appendix A: Glossary of Terms

Guillain-Barré Syndrome (GBS): A rare autoimmune disorder where the immune system attacks peripheral nerves, leading to muscle weakness, numbness, and potentially paralysis.

- Acute Inflammatory Demyelinating Polyneuropathy (AIDP): The most common form of GBS, characterized by the loss of the myelin sheath around peripheral nerves.

- Acute Motor Axonal Neuropathy (AMAN): A variant of GBS involving damage to the axons of peripheral nerves rather than the myelin sheath.

- Acute Motor and Sensory Axonal Neuropathy (AMSAN): A severe variant of GBS affecting both motor and sensory nerves.

- Miller Fisher Syndrome (MFS): A rare GBS variant marked by ataxia, ophthalmoplegia, and areflexia.

- Myelin: The fatty insulating sheath around nerve fibers that facilitates electrical impulse conduction.

Appendix B: Resources for Families

- National Institute of Neurological Disorders and Stroke (NINDS): Provides comprehensive information on GBS, including treatment options and research updates. Website: www.ninds.nih.gov

- The GBS|CIDP Foundation International: A worldwide association devoted to GBS and chronic inflammatory demyelinating polyneuropathy (CIDP) study, education, and support. Website: www.gbs-cidp.org

- What are the potential causes of my child's Guillain-Barré Syndrome?

- Which long-term and short-term treatment options are available?

- How can we manage symptoms and support recovery at home?

- What should we expect in terms of recovery timelines and outcomes?

- Are there any specific therapies or interventions that could aid in recovery?

- How can we monitor for complications and know when to seek emergency care?

Appendix D: Support Groups and Online Communities

- Inspire Community for Guillain-Barré Syndrome: An online forum where users can engage in discussions, ask questions, and receive support from peers. Website: www.inspire.com/groups/

- The GBS|CIDP Foundation International Forums: A place to find information, support, and community from others facing similar challenges. Website: forum.gbs-cidp.org/

Appendix E: Checklist for Managing GBS

- Before Diagnosis:
    - Record symptoms and their progression.
    - Note any recent infections or vaccinations.
    - Document any changes in mobility or sensation.
- After Diagnosis:
    - Follow the treatment plan as prescribed.
    - Attend all recommended therapy and follow-up appointments.
    - Note all symptoms, drugs, and adverse effects in a journal.
- Home Management:

- Implement necessary home modifications for accessibility.
  - Coordinate with healthcare providers for home care needs.
  - Engage in prescribed physical therapy and exercises.
- Emotional and Social Support:
  - Join community groups for practical and emotional advice.
  - Openly discuss your needs and challenges with family and friends.
  - Consider professional counseling if needed.

These appendices provide essential information and resources to support families dealing with Guillain-Barré Syndrome, offering guidance, connections, and practical tools to aid in managing the condition and navigating the recovery process.

About the Author

Dr. Travis R. Hill is a neurologist with vast pediatric care experience, specializing in tough neurological diseases like Guillain-Barré Syndrome (GBS). His clinical and scientific expertise motivated his commitment to aiding families through tough diagnoses. In his book, From Diagnosis to Recovery: A Parent's Survival Guide to Support Guillain-Barré Syndrome in Children, Dr. Hill blends medical information with compassionate guidance to empower parents battling GBS. Beyond his publications, he is an active instructor and contributor to medical education, dedicated to improving patient treatment and furthering understanding of neurological illnesses.

Thank you for reading this book. Your journey through this book is greatly appreciated. Please think about writing a review if this book was helpful. Your feedback helps other people find the support they need. Thanks for your support and kindness!

www.ingramcontent.com/pod-product-compliance
Lightning Source LLC
Chambersburg PA
CBHW070806250726
48662CB00004B/2009